EVENING PRIMROSE OIL

ITS AMAZING NUTRIENTS AND THE HEALTH BENEFITS THEY CAN GIVE YOU

by Dr. Richard A. Passwater

Keats Publishing, Inc.   New Canaan, Connecticut

Evening Primrose Oil is not intended as medical advice. Its intention is solely informational and educational. Please consult a medical or health professional should the need for one be warranted.

INTRODUCING EVENING PRIMROSE OIL

Once Evening Primrose was known chiefly for its beauty. A few knew of its healing powers as an herb, but all in all, not much attention has been paid to this lovely plant.

There are several varieties of the Evening Primrose, all being classified of the Onagraceae family (genus Primula). The most common varieties beautifying North America are Oenothera biennis, Oenothera caespitosa and Oenothera hookeri. Of course, most people would more easily recognize one of the common names such as King's Cure-all, sandlily, rockrose, hooker, sun drop, night willow herb, coffee plant, fever plant, scurvish, scabish, cabish, German ranpion, large ranpion, gumbo primrose, tree primrose, etc.

Perhaps the reason it has so many common names is that varieties grow throughout North America along streams and roadsides as border plants and in the high deserts more as a "field plant." It grows from sea level to 9000 feet above sea level.

Jack Challem, author of *What Herbs Are All About* (New Canaan, CT: Keats Publishing, Inc. 1980) describes the white-tufted Evening Primrose as a delicately petaled, large-flowered (3" diameter) plant with a light-green vein running down the centers of the lance-shaped leaves. Although some varieties are shorter, the plants are generally two to five feet tall. Challem recollects seeing the Evening Primrose in bloom for the first time. "They looked at first like tissue paper strewn across the desert. I had to stop because it looked like someone had littered the desert. . . ." He adds, "The delicate flowers generally last one night and wither to a pinkish color. They bloom in the evening and are pollinated by night-flying insects."

The white-tufted Evening Primrose produces flowers ranging from white to bright yellow, while other varieties produce red or lavender blooms. The plants are biennials requiring two years to bloom, after which they die in the fall.

The Pilgrims learned of the medicinal properties of the Evening Primrose from the Indians. The Evening Primrose was quickly exported to England where it soon became known as "King's Cure-all."

The Indians used whole-plant extracts of the Evening Primrose externally to heal wounds and soothe skin inflammations and eruptions. They used it internally to control coughs and infections.

Chief Two-Trees of the Cherokee nation, who has studied with several medicine men, reports that Evening Primrose is used to lessen spasms, as a sedative, pain killer, diuretic and a mild astringent. The root is used for making a cough syrup that is especially effective against whooping cough, asthmatic cough and tuberculosis cough. The sedative effect varies with the species and with the person. M. Moore suggests that this effect is due to the potassium nitrate found in all parts of the plant.[1]

The Evening Primrose today is desired not as an herb, but as the only known substantial source of a nutrient which is the focus of much current research.

Just at the time of greatest need, scientists have found that the oil of the Evening Primrose seed is rich in a rare nutrient that can help alleviate many health problems ranging from heart disease to arthritis to skin disorders. Research indicates furthermore that Evening Primrose Oil may be effective as part of any program to lose weight or to overcome alcoholism or schizophrenia.

The rare nutrient found in Evening Primrose Oil is *gamma-linolenic acid* (GLA)—by far the richest source, the oil is 9 percent GLA. (Incidentally, do not confuse GLA with linoleic acid or the common form of linolenic acid, which is the ineffective alpha-linolenic acid or ALA.) GLA is essential to good health because it is needed in order for the body to make a family of hormone-like compounds that control every organ in the body. These compounds especially affect the heart and circulation, skin and defense mechanism against disease. The members of this vital family of compounds are called *prosta-glandins* (PGs). Anyone having a deficiency of GLA will also have a shortage of PGs, resulting in impaired health. The nutritional optimization of PG is a revolutionary breakthrough in health care.

Even though your doctor may have prescribed Evening Primrose Oil as a dietary supplement, it is not a drug. It does not force your body to do or make anything. The extra GLA made available in your diet allows your body to make all the PGs needed for health. The roles of Evening Primrose Oil are both that of a nutrient and that of a remedial dietetic.

Evening Primrose Oil has:

- **lowered weight in the overweight without dieting**
- **lowered blood cholesterol**
- **lowered blood pressure to normal**
- **healed or improved eczema**
- **stopped rheumatoid arthritis in moderate cases**
- **normalized saliva and tear production**
- **relieved premenstrual pain**
- **slowed progression of multiple sclerosis**
- **improved acne when taken with zinc**
- **improved behavior and function of hyperactive children**
- **improved fingernails**
- **alleviated hangovers**

All of the above have been done with *people*. Evening Primrose Oil has also been found to do the following in laboratory animals:

- **slowed the rate of growth of breast cancer**
- **reduced the risk of thrombosis**
- **prevented the development of arthritis**

Clinical trials with people are planned for these.

GLA—A KEY NUTRIENT

GLA (gamma-linolenic acid) has achieved recognition in nutrition only recently. Previously it was believed that everyone could make their own GLA from an essential fatty acid called linoleic acid. Now we have learned that GLA is not being adequately formed in many people, resulting in major health problems.

Essential fatty acids (EFAs) are the simplest compounds that can be used for manufacturing other compounds in the body. EFAs are essential to the diet because they themselves cannot be manufactured in the body. Their importance is that they make other needed compounds, such as prostaglandins and thromboxanes. On the other hand, EFAs are useless unless they can be converted to other compounds.

While it is true that all essential fatty acids are polyunsaturated fatty acid, not many polyunsaturated fatty acids are essential to the diet. In fact, scientists now feel that *only* linoleic acid is a dietary essential. The body can make other vital fatty acids as needed provided it is well nourished with vitamins and minerals.

The EFAs are very much like a vitamin. Their absence causes deficiency diseases, just as a vitamin deficiency would. Before the EFAs were isolated and identified as fatty acids, they were actually thought to be a vitamin by researchers. The designation "vitamin F" was used during the early research (the term is obsolete now).

The symptoms noted in animals deficient in EFA include:

- **hair loss**
- **painful, swollen joints**
- **dry, scaly skin**
- **irritability**
- **lethargy**
- **infertility**
- **infections**
- **liver problems**
- **poor tissue structure**

These symptoms appear in humans as well, but few physicians think in terms of EFA deficiency: after all, we eat too much fat and food tables tell us that the "average person" consumes more than enough EFA. Until recently, it was not realized that factors in the typical diet could block GLA formation in the body. And it is the GLA and the resulting prostaglandins (PGs) that are important to health. EFA is just a starting point.

Another problem is that many people are deficient in the vitamins and minerals needed to finish the job of GLA and PG production. The above symptoms of EFA deficiency are similar to those of vitamin B6 deficiency and aging, both of which effect the production of GLA. Let's look at this more closely.

We can make GLA in our bodies out of the essential fatty acid *cis*-linoleic acid—provided that the reaction is not blocked by *trans*-linoleic acid (cis- and trans- refer to the arrangement of the atoms in the compound) or deficiencies of vitamin B6, zinc, magnesium or insulin. We *can* make GLA in our bodies, but the question is: Can we make enough GLA fast enough for optimum health? The answer for many people is "No" due to genetic limitations, nutrient deficiencies or blockage by other dietary factors.

So many people must depend on their diets to get optimal amounts of GLA. Evening Primrose Oil is an ideal way of obtaining GLA for two reasons; first, it is rich in GLA, and second, it is free of blocking agents.

There is a great biological difference caused by the very small structural difference between the two forms called "cis-" and "trans-." Trans-fatty acids differ from the naturally occurring cis-fatty acids in the manner in which they become incorporated into membranes of cells, thus affecting their function.[2] Also trans-fatty acids are incorporated differently into triglycerides and phospholipids. More importantly, trans-fatty acids greatly affect the utilization of EFA. Thus, trans-linoleic acid (tLA) blocks the utilization of cis-linoleic acid (cLA). The presence of trans-fatty acids in the diet increases the EFA requirement and aggravates the symptoms of EFA deficiency.[3]

The "cis-" form occurs in nature, while with few exceptions the "trans-" form is only made by man. Trans-fatty acids are widely distributed in the diet because processed vegetable oils are used in a vast variety of foods. Vegetable oils contain generous amounts of cis-polyunsaturated fatty acids. However, commercial processing to improve stability and odor converts a substantial amount of the cis-polyunsaturated fatty acids to

Important Polyunsaturated Fatty Acid Content of the Major Oils

Oil	cis-linoleic (cLA)	gamma-linolenic (GLA)	Blocking Fats
Evening Primrose	73%	9%	18%
Safflower	73%	—	27%
Corn	57%	—	43%
Sunflower	58%	—	42%
Soybean	51%	—	49%
Peanut	29%	—	71%
Olive	8%	—	92%
Coconut	2%	—	98%

GLA and PG Production

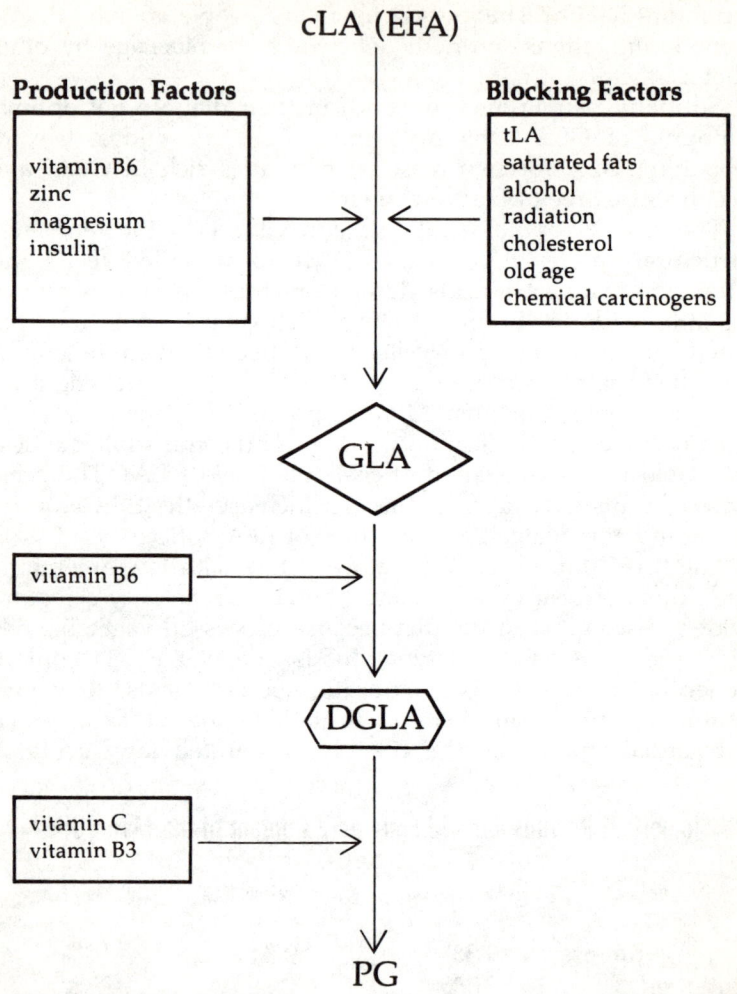

cLA (EFA)

Production Factors

vitamin B6
zinc
magnesium
insulin

Blocking Factors

tLA
saturated fats
alcohol
radiation
cholesterol
old age
chemical carcinogens

GLA

vitamin B6

DGLA

vitamin C
vitamin B3

PG

Shown are nutrient deficiencies and blocking factors which interfere with the body's production of GLA which is needed for the production of prostaglandins. PG regulates all organs and cells thus affecting the health of the body in many ways. When cLA is blocked, then you must get your GLA from the diet so that you can make optimal amounts of PG.

trans-polyunsaturated fatty acid. When vegetable or seed oils are hydrogenated to improve consistency and stability in producing margarine, not only are saturated fatty acids formed, but trans-polyunsaturated fatty acids are produced in great quantity. As an example, stick margarine contains from 25 to 35 percent trans-fatty acids, tub margarine 15 to 25 percent, shortening 20 to 30 percent, and salad oils 0 to 15 percent.[3]

To make a long story short, the typical American diet blocks the utilization of cLA. Estimates of cLA intake are too high because both cLA and tLA are lumped together. A large percentage of the cLA that is in the diet is useless because of the blocking fats or deficiencies in vitamin B6, zinc and magnesium. GLA bypasses these problems. Adding Evening Primrose Oil to the diet is a prudent step.

PROSTAGLANDINS—THE HEALTH CONTROLLERS

All of the chemistry presented so far establishes that we need gamma-linolenic acid in the diet. Even though the typical diet contains too much fat, not enough of the essential fatty acid cis-linoleic acid is converted to GLA.

The reason that we need the body well stocked with GLA is so that the body can make as much PG as it needs. The various human PGs are not readily obtainable in the diet, and if they were, since they are complex molecules, they would mostly be destroyed by the digestive process. Therefore, we should fortify our body's own production of GLA to assure optimal levels of PG.

Why?

• Because PGs control a multitude of essential functions in the body—such seemingly unrelated disorders as heart attacks, high blood pressure, arthritis, menstrual cramps, allergies, asthma, migraine headaches, fertility, glaucoma and, perhaps, cancer.

• Because PGs are not stored. Every tissue makes PG as needed. Their effect is very brief because they are quickly inactivated by enzymes. Some organ systems depend on a balance of PGs which act in opposite ways.

In recent years scientists have learned of the functions of approximately twenty different PGs. Of them, those of the families designated as E family and F family are the most important. They are abbreviated for convenience as PGE and PGF. One other PG family is of particular interest, that of the 'I' family. One member of the PGI family, PGI_2, often called "prostacyclin," is a particularly potent cellular regulator and anti-clotting agent. The most interesting family though, is PGE, and the most marvelous member of this family is PGE_1.

The subscripts refer to the EFA used as the starting point in its production. The PG series made from GLA are designated by the subscript 1. The PG series made from arachidonic acid (AA) are designated by the subscript 2, and the series from eicosapentaenoic acid (EPA) by the subscript 3. The biological differences between the three series seems to be dependent soley on the differences in the number of double bonds in the precursor polyunsaturated fatty acid.

It seems that PGs made from GLA and EPA have desirable functions that are often held in check by PGs from AA. PGE_1 and PGE_3 are protective against heart attacks caused by blood clot. PGE_1, PGE_3 and PGI_2 keep the blood platelets from sticking together, but PGE_2 promotes platelet aggregation (the first step in clotting).[4] A balance of PGE_1 and PGE_3 versus PGE_2 thus maintains the proper clotting mechanism. However, a shortage of PGE_1 or PGE_3 or an excess of PGE_2 will increase the tendency to form   heart attack-causing blood clots in the coronary arteries.

A *balance* of the appropriate fatty acids in the diet is required to maintain a proper clotting mechanism. Unfortunately, many people eat too much AA and tLA and not enough GLA, cLA and EPA.

In general, PGs of the E family and F family produce contrasting effects, and in some instances PGE_1 and PGE_2 have opposing actions.[5] PGE_1 is an effective inhibitor of blood clotting, while in contrast, PGE_2 accelerates blood clotting.[6] PGE_1 has a diuretic action, whereas PGE_2 causes the kidneys to retain salt, and thus increases water retention. Thus, PGE_2 has been implicated as a possible factor in high blood pressure.[7]

Dr. David Horrobin of the Institute for Innovative Medicine in Montreal has been the foremost researcher in the relationships between cLA, GLA and PG production. Dr. Horrobin stated in the medical literature, "The level of PGE_1 is of crucial importance to the body. A fall in the level of PGE_1 will lead to a potentially catastrophic series of untoward consequences including increased vascular reactivity, enhanced [blood clotting], elevated cholesterol production, [diabetic-like changes in insulin release], enhanced risk of auto-immune disease, enhanced release of AA, enhanced risk of inflammatory disorders and susceptibility to depression."[8]

PGE_1 is necessary for normal function of the T-cells of the immune system (these cells reject foreign bodies). In cell cultures, PGE_1 reduced the rate of cell division in a malignant tissue and restored cell normality. PGE_1 reduces the release of inflammation-causing lysosomes, and slows the formation of inflammation-producing PGE_2 by blocking AA release from storage. It has prevented arthritis in rats and auto-immune disease in mice.

PGE_1 affects the release of compounds from nerve cells that transmit nerve impulses; it also seems to regulate calcium movement in cells.

PGE_1 has many more functions that affect several disease processes, as we shall now see.

HEART DISEASE AND EVENING PRIMROSE OIL

What relationship could this ubiquitous delicate flower, the Evening Primrose, have to heart health? The relationship is not that of medicine known only to the esoteric. So many people have messed up their diets that a nutrient uniquely found in the seed of the Evening Primrose is widely required to restore balance and thus heart health.

Most Western diets today have two flaws. One flaw is that they are deficient in some nutrients and the second is that they have too much of other nutrients. Modern Western diets have insufficient quantities of the essential fatty acid (EFA), cis-linoleic acid (cLA) and certain vitamins (including vitamins B6, C and E) and minerals (including magnesium and selenium). Today's typical diets also contain fats, called trans-fats, that block the utilization of cLA. These dietary flaws hamper the production of prostaglandins, required for heart and circulatory system health.

Heart Attacks: Heart attacks are caused by insufficient blood reaching the heart or a serious irregularity in the heart beat. The problem of insufficient blood can be caused by clots in a coronary artery, resulting in blocked blood flow, or by spasms in an artery. Fat and cholesterol-containing deposits contribute to clot formation.

When blood supply through a coronary artery is insufficient, the tissue fed by that artery dies. If the area of destroyed heart tissue is small, the damage is not serious and tough fibrous "scar" tissue patches over the damage. Recovery can be complete.

The formation of a clot in a coronary artery is called "coronary thrombosis" and the resultant death of heart tissue is called "myocardial infarction."

Preventing Clot-Type of Heart Attacks: Blood is normally a slippery fluid. If we were to cut ourselves, however, all of our blood could run out unless something would plug the wound. The body does this by causing the blood to clot. Under the conditions of a wound, blood platelets (plate-like components in blood about one-half the size of red blood cells) adhere together to initiate the clotting procedure.

The tendency for blood to clot is measured by an index called the "platelet adhesion index." A healthy person would typically have a platelet adhesion index near 20. This means that their blood is not sticky. The measurement is made by flowing blood over glass beads in an instrument. The number 20 indicates that 20 percent of the platelets stuck to the beads. Measurements taken of recent heart attack victims are as high as 90. Such blood is very prone to clotting.

Normally, artery walls make prostacyclin (PGI_2) which prevents the platelets from sticking to each other or to artery walls. However, arteries damaged by fat and cholesterol deposits, high blood pressure, or injury do not make adequate amounts of PGI_2. Platelet adhesion to cholesterol deposits results in rapid build up of a clot, which can block the blood flow.

As we have seen, PGE_1 and PGE_3 can both reduce blood platelet adhesion. The dietary intake of GLA in Evening Primrose Oil is an important aid in keeping blood slippery and preventing clotting. Vitamin E and fish oils (EPA) also aid in restoring proper blood slipperiness.

Thus, even if you have cholesterol deposits in your arteries, there is no need to have a heart attack. Coronaries were un-known until the turn of the century, when food processing began refining vitamins B6 and E, and the mineral magnesium out of the food supply. Heart attacks became epidemic after 1920 when man-made trans-fats which block cLA utilization were introduced to the food supply. The main problem is not the deposits, but sticky blood.

Evening Primrose Oil bypasses this problem by providing GLA and making PGE_1, which keeps your blood slippery.

Preventing Spasm-Type Heart Attacks: There is a case when normal blood slipperiness will not be enough to protect you. Let's consider artery construction for a moment to see why.

Arteries have a built-in defense mechanism against a very strong shock. The artery walls can constrict tightly to shut off blood flow if they are cut during severe injury. However, sometimes the artery walls are stimulated to contract by emo-tional shock or stress. Artery spasms are more apt to occur in conjunction with dietary imbalances such as magnesium defi-ciency or available cLA deficiency.

Spasm-type heart attacks were thought to be rare a few years ago. An Italian research team found that at least 20 percent of all fatal heart attacks were artery spasms. New testing tech-niques were developed that indicate that a larger percentage—perhaps the majority—of fatal heart attacks are caused by artery spasms.

Artery spasms are usually fatal only when the constricting artery is already partially blocked by cholesterol and fat depos-its. Of course, what started investigators into this direction of research were the heart attacks observed in young people with deposit-free arteries.

The mechanism involved in spasm-type heart attack is as follows. Stress causes the nerves to release chemicals which in turn cause the arteries to constrict. The reduced blood supply also reduces the oxygen available to the artery muscle. If this oxygen reduction is mild, the artery relaxes. However, if the oxygen supply is severely reduced, the muscle goes into spasms.

Keep in mind that cigarette smokers already have reduced available oxygen, and smokers have greater risk for the spasm to develop rather than artery relaxation. Stress and smoking are a killing combination.

During artery spasm, PGI_2 is not released and PGE_2 may be released. As a result blood platelets clump together and adhere to the artery wall to form a more lasting seal. This is a key point. It takes two to three hours for permanent heart tissue change to occur. The heart tissue will not die if the blood shortage is only temporary. If the artery spasm can be relaxed in a short time, no permanent damage will occur. However, if the spasm lasts sufficiently long, a blood clot occurs which makes a seal lasting long enough to cause tissue death.

Other Heart Problems Are Related: The partially blocked artery increases the probability of heart damage by either clot formation or arterial spasm. If the area of the heart affected is the "pacemaker" that controls heart beat, an irregular beat can result that is too weak to pump blood adequately. This grossly irregular beat is called ventricular fibrillation. Ventricular fibrillation can have other causes besides infarction (tissue death).

Angina pectoris is the severe chest pain that develops during exertion or stress. The partially clogged arteries can supply sufficient blood to meet heart oxygen needs only when the person is resting. Movement or emotional stress creates a greater oxygen demand which cannot be met. The result is that the heart releases chemicals that cause pain and warn the person to slow down. A continued oxygen shortage can lead to artery spasm and then tissue damage.

Dilation of the coronary arteries increases blood flow thus quenching the pain. Nitroglycerin dilates arteries, and so does PGE_1. Many have found that increased dietary GLA reduces their need for nitroglycerin and can greatly reduce the number and severity of their angina attacks.

Evening Primrose Oil has a lot to offer the heart patient. However, it is not a drug and it doesn't work immediately during a heart attack. Evening Primrose Oil does offer the angina patient partial relief in a relatively short time, however.[9]

Typical effective supplement protocol for heart disease that has also lowered blood cholesterol, and helped normalize body weight has been three to four 500 milligram Evening Primrose Oil capsules in the morning with an equal amount taken in the evening.[10]

Vitamin E should also be considered for use in a strategy against heart disease. Vitamin E increases the formation of prostacyclin (PGI_2), thus lowering blood platelet adhesion. There are also reports that vitamin E increases the "good" cholesterol carrier, called high density lipoprotein (HDL), that is protective against heart disease.

Evening Primrose Oil and Blood Cholesterol Levels

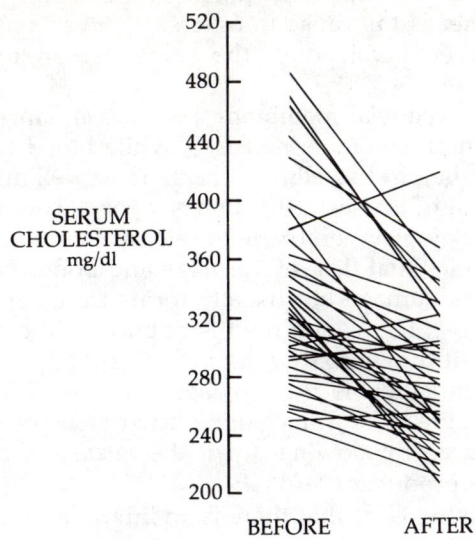

SERUM CHOLESTEROL mg/dl

BEFORE   AFTER

Changes in blood cholesterol levels in individuals who took four to six capsules of Evening Primrose Oil for periods of two to twelve months. (*Courtesy of Dr. D. Horrobin*)

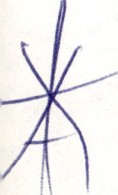

ARTHRITIS

Arthritis lessens the quality of life for millions of people. Often the pain can be controlled, but the damage to the bone joint continues until mobility is lost. There are two common types of arthritis. Evening Primrose Oil has been shown to be effective against rheumatoid arthritis; at this writing it has not been tried against osteoarthritis, a "wear and tear" type of damage.

Rheumatoid arthritis begins as an inflammation in the membrane that produces the fluid that lubricates bone joints. This membrane is called the synovial membrane. The cause of the inflammation is not certain, but many medical researchers feel that the body's immune system mistakenly attacks the joints. Diet and stress have also been suggested as being responsible for initiating the inflammation, and it's possibile that all three are involved. Perhaps one causes arthritis in some people, while another is the cause in others. It's even possible that all three must be involved in the same person to initiate the inflammation.

When the synovial membrane becomes inflamed, the blood supply to the membrane increases, white blood cells gather in the membrane, and swelling occurs. The swelling can become severe enough to push the bones apart. The inflammation causes the synovial membrane to release chemicals called lysosomal enzymes that destroy cartilage and bone. The body tries to repair this damage but usually forms irregular patches and rough bumps. These outgrowths aggravate the problem and decrease joint function.

The inflammation is brought about by the 2 series prostaglandins produced from arachidonic acid (AA). The inflammation can be reduced by slowing down the release of stored AA or slowing the production of PGE_2.

It is becoming clear that there is an interrelationship between PG, vitamin E, aspirin and steroid drugs. The interrelationship can be explained by looking at the pathways for using EFA. So far we have concentrated on how EFA is made into PG. However, there is another important pathway wherein EFA produces a particularly nasty compound called "leukotrienes." Leukotrienes do have a positive function. They are desirable during wound healing. However, they can be released under other conditions that can be bothersome. Poorly controlled leukotriene production is suspected of causing such unpleasant effects as arthritic inflammation and the painful breast lumps of cystic mastitis. Leukotrienes are formed from arachidonic acid (AA). AA can be converted to PG or leukotriene. Excesses of either PGE_2 or leukotriene can be a problem. PGE_2 can lead to unwanted blood clotting, pain or fever depending on the tissues in which it is produced. Aspirin can reduce the production of PGE_2. This explains how aspirin reduces pain and fever, and how it can under certain conditions reduce the risk of a clot forming in the coronary artery. This also explains how aspirin has the undesirable side effects of gastrointestinal bleeding. It also explains why aspirin reduces the pain of arthritis with little effect on inflammation.

Dr. David Cornwell of Ohio State has elucidated the mechanism of leukotriene production. Leukotriene production can be brought under control by slowing the release of AA from storage or by slowing the conversion of AA to leukotriene with vitamin E.

Drugs such as corticosteroids or indomethacin act on pain and inflammation by slowing AA release from storage. Thus both PGE_2 and leukotriene production are slowed, which in turn controls both pain and inflammation. Unfortunately, these drugs also have serious drawbacks. Neither aspirin nor steroids affect the long term course of arthritis because they block the production of the desirable PGE_1. However, there is a better way to slow AA release from storage.

The preferred way to control AA release from storage is by PGE_1. If adequate GLA is available, then PGE_1 can be produced to balance PGE_2 and also control AA release. It is always preferable to utilize natural body compounds to regulate the body rather than to use synthetic drugs, such as aspirin or indomethacin, if the same degree of control can be achieved.

Fairly strong evidence exists that in some individuals at least the inflammation is caused or aggravated by food allergies. Foods of the nightshade family (including potatoes, tomatoes, peppers, paprika and eggplant) and wheat are particularly suspect for such food allergies.

If you are interested in checking to see if you are the victim of food allergy, you could consider the merits of removing the possible offenders for three months. You might wish to first remove all nightshade plants, and if that doesn't help, add them back and then remove all wheat products.

Dr. David Horrobin of Montreal explains that in some patients such a nutritional approach alone may be adequate, while in others, additional support from drugs may be necessary.[11]

Evening Primrose Oil is effective in controlling rheumatoid arthritis in a substantial number of patients.[12] However, three factors should be noted. First, Evening Primrose Oil does not benefit patients receiving more than trivial doses of steroids, indomethacin-like or aspirin-like drugs. This is because they have conflicting action on PGE_1. However, Evening Primrose Oil can be taken and then the drug dosage reduced after one to three months.

Second, the benefits of Evening Primrose Oil do not become apparent for one to three months. Some patients experience a transient setback during the first week or two, although they do best in the long run.

Third, there is preliminary evidence that the disease may be actually *halted* in some patients, as opposed to the action of the drugs.[11] Of course, it would be too much to expect reversal of pre-existing damage.

Evening Primrose Oil has been helpful in many patients at the three to four gram level of intake. This represents three to four 500 milligram capsules taken at both morning and evening. Other dietary deficiencies should be corrected. This is especially true of vitamins B6, C, E and pantothenic acid.

WEIGHT CONTROL

Some "overweight" people eat more food than normal weight people. On the other hand a great many "fat" people eat no more—and even less—than "thin" people. "But I eat like a bird" is often exclaimed by the frustrated perennial dieter. Of course, if you eat more calories than you burn, you will put on fat. However, the key is that some people do not burn their calories as easily as others.

In the past, this has been explained away as being due to differences in basal metabolism (the energy needed just to keep the body alive). This basic energy-burning rate is dependent on genetics, exercise level and hormonal relationships. Now we know of a separate mechanism that burns calories and helps determine who's thin and who's fat.

Thin people seem to have a well-functioning mechanism to burn off extra calories, whereas fat people have a faulty mechanism—or the mechanism is poorly developed. The body has a special tissue of brown fat located in the back of the neck and along the backbone. The brown coloration is due to the high concentration of cellular energy-producing (fat burning) units called mitochondria. The brown fat burns calories not to produce energy for body movement, but solely for heat. One role of brown fat is weight stabilization, another is adaptation to cold weather.

Appetite control is centered in a region of the brain called the ventromedial hypothalamus. Appetite regulation utilizes a feedback mechanism that senses insulin and amino acid content of the blood. It is believed that the ventromedial hypothalamus can switch on the brown fat tissue whenever excess calories are consumed. Obese persons may either have a faulty "switch" or they may have insufficient brown fat.

Before the brown fat mechanism was elucidated, many investigators were seeking the "mechanism X". It was obvious that an unknown mechanism existed, but the mechanism was so different from what was expected that it was overlooked. The role of brown fat in weight regulation was more or less uncovered by research into cold adaptation.

The "brown fat" discovery was made by several researchers including Dr. David G. Nicholls of the University of Dundee, Scotland; Dr. Jean Himms-Hagen of the University of Ottawa; Dr. Michael Stock of St. George's Hospital medical school in London; and Dr. George Bray of the University of California at Los Angeles.

The gamma-linolenic acid (GLA) content of Evening Primrose Oil has a stimulating effect on brown fat tissue. GLA forms certain prostaglandins that accelerate the mitochondria activity in the brown fat.

A large clinical trial in Heidelberg, West Germany, demonstrated that the fatter people were the less polyunsaturated fatty acids they had in the body, and the converse.[13] Those with high polyunsaturated fatty acid content tended to be of normal weight. Dr. David Horrobin of Montreal postulates that fat people may be suffering from a polyunsaturated fatty acid deficiency. Dr. Horrobin has found that GLA is remarkably effective in causing weight loss, and that Evening Primrose Oil is a particularly valuable dietary component in those who want to lose weight.[14]

In a study by Dr. K.S. Vaddadi and Dr. David Horrobin, Evening Primrose Oil lowered body weight in about half of those who were more than 10 percent overweight. *The effect was achieved without conscious dieting*, although those who lost weight said that they spontaneously felt less hungry.[14]

Keep in mind that body fat is also determined by what you eat and when you eat, as well as how much you eat. Good

Evening Primrose Oil and Weight Normalization

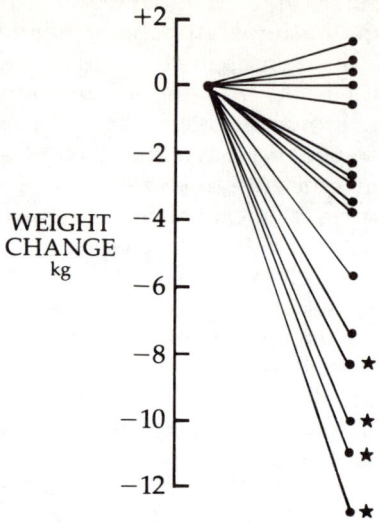

Changes in weight in 16 individuals who were more than 10% of their ideal body weight who took evening primrose oil for 6 to 8 weeks. The starred individuals took eight capsules per day while the others took four capsules per day. No weight changes occurred in 22 individuals who were within 10% of their ideal body weight. (*courtesy of Dr. David Horrobin*)

quality foods produce less body fat than junk foods because of their effect on insulin release.[15]

Never try to crash diet. The results are short term. Adjust your eating behavior to good nutritional foods, spaced into frequent small meals, prior to your energy needs. Lose a pound or two a week and you have a better chance to keep it off.

Balance your diet and take a vitamin and mineral supplement to ensure that you maintain adequate nourishment even though your food quality may be reduced.

Consider the beneficial effect of Evening Primrose Oil on brown fat tissue and weight normalization.

CANCER AND IMMUNITY

It has now become obvious that what you eat helps your body fight off cancer. Deficiencies of any of the major antioxidant nutrients (vitamins A, C and E plus the mineral selenium) have been shown to increase susceptibility to cancer in man and other animals.[16,17] Dietary supplements of these same antioxidant nutrients have been shown to increase resistance to cancer.

Several biochemical mechanisms are involved in the protective roles of the antioxidant nutrients, but the most important is the stimulation of the immune response. Now we have learned that we have a new ally in our natural defense against cancer. The hormone-like PGs affect the immune system. One PG, made from the gamma-linolenic acid found in Evening Primrose Oil, stimulates the T-cells of the immune system and, amazingly, *reverts cancer cells back to normal cells in test tube experiments.*

This compound, called PGE, has been extensively discussed throughout this booklet. PGE_1 is required for the T-cells (T-lymphocytes) of the immune system to attack a cancer. In fact, PGE_1 plays a major role in the regulation of thymus gland development, as well as in T-cell function.

T-cells play a critical role in cellular immunity. A deficiency in GLA, vitamin C, vitamin B6 or zinc leads to inadequate PGE_1 production and thus defective T-cell function.[18]

Thus, these nutrients are required in optimal quantities to maintain optimal immunity.

The immune system is our last line of defense against cancer. Our first line of defense is our liver which can detoxify cancer-causing chemicals. Our second line of defense is the cell membrane which controls cell nourishment and protects cells against invasion by cancer-causing chemicals.

Many scientists believe that healthy people routinely develop pre-cancerous cells that are destroyed by the immune system before they can form a full-fledged cancer. Strengthening of the immune system to prevent—and perhaps overcome—cancer is not a new strategy. However, reversing cancer cells back to normal cells is a new approach.

Dr. David Horrobin writes in *Medical Hypothesis*:

> Cancer therapy is dominated by the idea that treatment must aim at destruction of cancer cells. The goal is to exploit some difference between the cancer cells and the normal cells which will allow the cancerous ones to be selective destroyed. The selectivity of current chemotherapy and radiation therapy, such as it is, depends on the idea that the already damaged regulatory functions of cancer cells can be totally disrupted more easily than those of normal cells. Since the purpose of these treatments is to produce damage, it is not surprising that they harm normal cells. It is thus not surprising that most cancer therapeutic agents are themselves carcinogens and vice versa. A more rational aim in cancer would be the normalization of cancer cells by techniques which will do no harm to normal tissues. I propose that we already have the necessary information to enable this to be carried out.

> Very little attention has been paid to the possibility of normalizing cancer cells. This is largely because of the dominant theme of research into the cause of cancer is that the disease is brought about by irreversible and uncontrollable mutation, probably within the nuclear DNA or possibly within one of the other nucleic acid pools such as that in the mitochondria. However, it is by no means clear that carcinogenic mutations can never be repaired, nor that irreversible mutations are necessarily uncontrollable, nor that mutation is always a necessary condition of cancer development. Indeed, several lines of evidence indicate that the idea of treating cancer by normalizing cancer cells is not completely unrealistic.[17]

Cancer cells are already defective and have a high rate of death. The cancer grows only because the proliferation rate exceeds the cell death rate. If proliferation can be controlled by normalizing cell function, then the already damaged cancer cells will die and the cancer will regress.

PGE_1 is one of the most potent natural agents which can induce cancer cell reversal.[19] Even genetic mutations can be kept in check and sometimes reversed by PGE_1.

Cancer cells produce excessive amounts of the 2 series PG and cannot make PGE_1.[18] Now there is evidence that PGE_1 together with thromboxane (TX_2), another important family of compounds made from cLA, AA and EPA, can reverse all the abnormalities common to cancer cells.

Dr. Horrobin has proposed that the critical step in cancer cell formation is the loss of the ability to make PGE_1 and/or TX_2. He believes that restoration of normal PGE_1 levels by providing GLA will be of value in reversing cancer growth.

In test tubes or cell cultures, human cells can be transformed to cancer cells by radiation or carcinogens. In the transformation process, the cells lose their ability to convert cLA into GLA, and hence to make PGE_1.[18,20,21] The malignant cells can be made normal by exposing them to PGE_1.[18,22,23]

The action of vitamin C might be enhanced by administering it with Evening Primrose Oil which would restore the responsiveness of the cells to vitamin C. Trials of the value of combined treatment with vitamin C and Evening Primrose Oil are now in progress at several centers.

PREMENSTRUAL PAIN, CYSTIC MASTITIS AND BRITTLE NAILS

Evening Primrose Oil corrects several problems of special interest to women. If for no other reason, this may make Evening Primrose Oil the best discovery of the century.

The pain of premenstrual tension is both physical and mental. Increased water retention swells tissues which results in abdominal pain and depression. Depression and irritability result from the brain swelling against the confinement of the skull.

The gradual increase in fluid can produce pain and mood change beginning from two to fourteen days before menstruation starts. Diuretics help reduce the build-up and bring some relief. However, care must be taken to assure an adequate intake of potassium and magnesium, which have a greater rate of loss from the body with the use of diuretics.

We can increase the effectiveness of the relief naturally without the need for diuretics.

Vitamin B6 has been very effective in about 70 percent of the women with premenstrual tension. Also vitamin E has helped many. But now we understand the interactions of vitamin B6, vitamin E, gamma-linolenic acid (GLA) and prostaglandins(PG). Vitamin B6 is needed for the conversion of cis-linoleic acid to the prostaglandin PGE_1. Vitamin E helps keep the nasty compounds called leukotrienes from being formed and encourages the production of the preferred PGE_1. GLA bypasses the problem of inefficient cis-linoleic acid conversion and also enhances PGE_1 production.

British studies have now found that Evening Primrose Oil, the natural source of GLA can relieve about 90 to 95 percent of women's premenstrual tension.[24] They have found that Evening Primrose Oil cures two-thirds of the women not helped by anything else, while another 20 percent were greatly improved.

The secret is not to wait until the discomfort begins but to take vitamin B6 and Evening Primrose Oil daily. Many have found that 50 milligrams of vitamin B6 and six 500 milligram capsules of Evening Primrose Oil daily are effective. The Evening Primrose Oil capsules should be divided into two or three doses during the day. Extremely difficult cases may need a total of eight 500 milligram capsules of Evening Primrose Oil and up to 200 milligrams of vitamin B6. Vitamin E is generally helpful in the 100 to 600 milligram range.

Evening Primrose Oil has also aided women with heavy and prolonged bleeding. Instead of a heavy blood loss for seven to ten days, their periods normalized to four or five days duration at normal blood loss.

The same protective regimen used for premenstrual tension would be effective for many women with heavy and prolonged periods. Relief should occur within two or three cycles. However, some cases will not respond and surgery to remove the fibroids may be required to relieve the problem.

The most common breast disease is cystic mastitis (also called benign breast disease of fibrocystic disease of the breast, mammary dysplasia, or fibrous mastopathy), which affects about 20 percent of premenopausal women. Often cysts (lumps) are tender and painful especially prior to menstrual flow; however, the larger percentage of cysts are not painful.

The cause of the cysts is thought to be an overproduction of the hormone prolactin, combined with a shortage of PGE_1. Evening Primrose Oil helps prevent cyst development and speedily removes existing lumps. This was discovered by accident while Evening Primrose Oil was being administered to large numbers of women for other reasons. The disappearance or softening of cysts occured within a two to four month period.

Vitamin E also helps this condition, as we saw in our discussion of the interrelationship of vitamin E and GLA. A "double-blind" study led by Dr. Robert S. London at the Johns Hopkins University School of Medicine and Sinai Hospital in Baltimore found that 85 percent of women with advanced cases of the disease responded within eight weeks to 600 milligrams of vitamin E daily. Forty percent of the women had a *complete disappearance* of the lumps.

The same regimen of Evening Primrose Oil, vitamin B6 and vitamin E, effective against premenstrual stress and heavy and prolonged bleeding, looks promising against cystic mastitis. Six to eight 500 milligram capsules of Evening Primrose Oil daily should, by itself, be effective for the vast majority of women. Stubborn cases may need the assist from the other vitamins.

Another surprising result of the research with Evening Primrose Oil is that brittle finger nails harden and become normal within about two to six weeks. This response is so consistent that it can be concluded that brittle nails are a newly recognized sign of essential fatty acid deficiency in humans. These findings have been published in the May 1981 issue of the *British Journal of Dermatology*. The benefit of this discovery is obvious to women, but also think about its potential use by doctors to diagnose essential fatty acid deficiency.

OTHER DISEASES

Other diseases are also responding to Evening Primrose Oil supplementation according to preliminary clinical results. Disease as diverse as diabetes, alcoholism, schizophrenia, multiple sclerosis, hyperactivity, infertility and eczema are among the many helped by Evening Primrose Oil. Although these diseases do not seem to be related in any way, they all involve a disturbance in prostaglandin balance. The gamma-linolenic acid naturally found in Evening Primrose Oil helps to restore the desired PG balance.

Diabetes: At this writing no definitive studies have been completed on Evening Primrose Oil and diabetes. However, a five-year study led by Dr. A. Houtsmuller found that diabetics on a diet rich in essential fatty acid had significantly less eye and heart disease than those on typical diets.[25]

The roles of PG and insulin are interrelated to the mineral zinc. PG helps zinc absorption and zinc aids the production of 1 series PG.[26] PGE_1 is able to enhance various actions of insulin. It is possible that some of the insulin resistance which occurs in diabetes could be due to insufficient PGE_1.

Alcoholism: Alcoholics tend to have elevated PGE_1 levels while drinking and then a crash to a very low PGE_1 level afterwards. This results in the "hangover" syndrome. (Although this is of little or no interest to health-minded readers, you may have friends that would be delighted to know that Evening Primrose Oil cures hangovers.)

PGE_1 affects calcium release which in turn affects nerve transmissions. There are many similarities between the "feminized" state of the chronic male alcoholic and men with chronic zinc or essential fatty acid deficiency. There are similarities between the congenital abnormalities associated with zinc deficiency and with the fetal alcohol syndrome. Part of the effect may be due to alcohol depletion of zinc, but another part may be that both lead to failure of normal PGE_1 production.[27,28] Thus there is an indication that PGE_1 may be a key determinant of mood and that some people may drink alcohol as a means of normalizing their brain level of PGE_1. If this is correct, then normalizing their PGE_1 level by nutritional means should reduce their craving for alcohol.

Drs. John Rotrosen and David Sagarnick of New York University have found that Evening Primrose Oil is very effective in preventing withdrawal symptoms in alcohol-addicted mice.

Schizophrenia: Schizophrenia is a biochemical disease in which sensual stimulations and thought processes become disordered. Schizophrenics do not have a "dual personality" or "split mind" as is so commonly stated. If the biochemistry of the nerve impulse transmission can be normalized, the person becomes normal.

In 1975, researchers at Guy Hospital in London found that blood platelets from schizophrenics completely failed to produce PGE_1. There is reason to believe that normalization of PGE_1 production can help schizophrenia.

There may indeed be several "causes" of schizophrenia, but these "causes" may only be different agitators of the real cause—abnormal PGE_1 production.

As Dr. David Horrobin writes in *The Lancet*:

"In recent years it has been suggested that the biological defect in schizophrenia may be related to excess dopamine (a compound involved in nerve transmission) activity, to production of an abnormal opioid or a normal opioid in excess, to a prostaglandin deficiency, to a hypersensitivity to wheat proteins, to an allergic phenomenon, to a defect in zinc metabolism, or to a pineal deficiency. . . . The various concepts are not mutually exclusive, but represent different aspects of the same problem. The final common path in schizophrenia may be a failure of formation and action of prostaglandins of the 1 series."[29]

Striking case histories have been reported in the medical literature. Dr. K.S. Vaddadi, Senior Registrar in Adult Psychiatry at Bootham Park Hospital in York, England reports the following:

"We have administered Evening Primrose Oil together with penicillin to six severe chronic schizophrenics inadequately controlled by phenothiazines: in all cases all other drug therapy was withdrawn. No patient has become worse during a 16-week period and in some the improvement has been striking."[30]

Patients who had been severely ill from twelve to twenty-one years in spite of treatment with several different drugs showed a dramatic improvement when oral penicillin was administered in combination with Evening Primrose Oil. (Penicillin is used because it stimulates PGE_1 production.)

Multiple Sclerosis: *The Multiple Sclerosis Diet Book* by Dr. Roy Swank touts the virtue of polyunsaturated fatty acids in controlling multiple sclerosis. The diet is controversial, but many other physicians are finding it beneficial.

Polyunsaturated fatty acids are not the main factor. PG formation from the essential fatty acid is the main factor. Better results could possibly come from adding the factors needed to convert cis-linolenic acid to the diet to make GLA, and by removing factors that block GLA formation.

Another approach is to supplement the diet with GLA from Evening Primrose Oil. There are about 3000 MS patients taking Evening Primrose Oil with good results.[31]

Research with laboratory animals preceded this development. In rats, there is a disease called experimental allergic encephalomyelitis which in some respects is very similar to human MS. Evening Primrose Oil has been found highly effective in preventing this disease.

As a result of these studies patients with MS have begun to take Evening Primrose Oil. The indications are that perhaps 15-20 percent of patients may be helped in a major way and another 15-20 percent in a minor way; 60-70 percent of patients are not helped and in no way is this a cure for the disease. However, in some patients, the improvements have been dramatic and it seems worthwhile to give the oil a trial in all patients. A suitable regime is to start with four capsules per day for three months, to increase this to eight capsules per day for a further three months and to twelve capsules per day for a further three months. If, after this time, there has been no improvement it is probably not worth continuing.

In England, a patients' organization called Action for Research on Multiple Sclerosis has accumulated evidence to suggest that Evening Primrose Oil slows down the progression of the disease.

Hyperactivity: A British group, Hyperactive Children's Support Group (HCSG), assembled information that led them to suspect that hyperactivity might be linked with a problem with PG. Their more than seventy branch chapters conducted an extensive survey profiling the characteristics of hyperactive children.

Dr. David Horrobin concurred and designed a therapeutic protocol. The preliminary results are encouraging. Dr. Horrobin says, "Studies have been initiated in several countries on the use of primrose oil in hyperactivity. About twenty children have been treated to date and there has been substantial benefit in about two thirds of them. Some of the responses have been dramatic. In one case a boy who had been threatened with expulsion from school because of his impossible behavior was put on primrose oil without the knowledge of the school authorities. After two weeks on GLA the teacher who was unaware of the treatment contacted the parents and said that in thirty years' experience she had never seen such a dramatic and abrupt change for the better in a child's behavior. Some children appear to do equally well no matter whether the oil is given by mouth or by rubbing into the skin. In others there is the distinct impression that skin absorption which will by-pass malabsorption problems may have a better effect."

I asked Dr. Horrobin how his observations fit in with those of Dr. Ben Feingold of the Kaiser Foundation Hospital-Permanent Medical Group in San Francisco. Dr. Horrobin replied, "Our findings dovetail very nicely. Feingold has described a large number of natural food substances and food additives which may precipitate symptoms in hyperactive children. These include natural salicylates, butylated hydroxytoluene (BHT), butylated hydroxyanisole (BHA), tartrazine and other colouring materials. Such materials do not, however, precipitate symptoms in normal children. The agents described by Feingold are almost all known inhibitors of conversion of EFAs to PGs or are chemically related to such known inhibitors. For other reasons my group investigated one of the worst offenders, tartrazine, in my laboratory some years ago. We found that it was an effective inhibitor of PG formation when EFA levels were very low but had little or no effect when EFA levels were high. This suggests the possibility that in children with normal EFA levels the materials will have no effect. The fact that they do have such dramatic effects in hyperactive children may indicate that in those children the levels of EFAs are unusually low."

The survey had uncovered the following four points that suggested EFA might be involved.

1. Hyperactive male children in HCSG outnumber females by about 3:1, a ratio which fits with surveys in North America. Male animals require a two to three-fold higher intake of EFAs than females in order to prevent signs of EFA deficiency. Therefore in any situation in which the supply of EFAs is marginal, males are likely to be affected much more substantially than females.
2. About two thirds of the children in HCSG appear to experience abnormal thirst. Thirst is one of the key features of EFA deficiency in animals.
3. Studies sponsored by HCSG have found low levels of zinc in the hair of many of their children. A lack of zinc will reduce formation of GLA from cLA and will block mobilization of DGLA.
4. HCSG have found that eczema, asthma and other features

of the atopic state are much commoner in hyperactive children than in normal ones. Such problems are associated with defective T-cell function which could be caused by lack of enough PGE.

5. HCSG have found that some of their children react badly to wheat products and/or milk. Both wheat and milk may give rise to opioids in the gut as product of partial digestion. Opioids have the capacity to block PGE formation from DGLA under certain conditions.

6. HCSG has many examples of families in which there is only one hyperactive child while other siblings eating exactly the same diet are normal. It is therefore unlikely that hyperactivity is associated with any obvious deficiency of dietary cLA. Hyperactive children could have a defect in EFA absorption which means that they may require much larger amounts of dietary EFAs than normal. Alternately they may have a defect preventing them from converting cLA normally to GLA.

Skin, Acne, and Eczema: Essential fatty acids are needed for healthy skin and hair. An EFA deficiency results in skin lesions, flaking dandruff, brittle nails and thinning hair. Correcting the diet by adding more EFA doesn't always work because the EFA may be blocked by trans-fatty acids or the person may not have adequate vitamins B6 and C, or the minerals magnesium and zinc in the diet. Evening Primrose Oil bypasses this problem by supplying the immediate PG-precursor GLA.

Evening Primrose Oil by itself has shown little effect on acne, but when given with zinc, it often produces striking improvement.

Research led by Dr. C.R. Lovell at the Department of Dermatology of the Royal Infirmary in Bristol, England has shown that Evening Primrose Oil significantly improved patients with severe atopic eczema. The double-blind, placebo-controlled clinical trial supported the thesis that an EFA abnormality was involved in the disease.

Dry Eyes and Mouth: Sjogren's syndrome (failure of saliva and tear gland function coupled with connective tissue disease) and sicca syndrome (failure of saliva and tear gland function without connective tissue disease) both respond to Evening Primrose Oil supplementation. These disorders can aggravate other body processes. Without adequate saliva, teeth are less cleansed and the gastrointestinal system is strained. Thus, relief of these problems by Evening Primrose Oil may prevent other disorders.

SUMMARY

A revolution in health care is unfolding due to our new understanding of the role of nutrition and prostaglandins. What has been discussed in this booklet is only the beginning of this revolution. Evening Primrose Oil provides us with a vital nutritional compound intermediate in PGE_1 production that bypasses many of the problems caused by modern Western diets.

REFERENCES

1 Moore, M. 1979. *Medicinal Herbs of the West* (74). University of New Mexico Press

Additional information can be found in herbalogy tests such as: Angier, B. 1978. *Field Guide to Medicinal Plants*. Harrisburg, PA: Stackpole Books

Coon, Nelson. 1963. *Using Plants for Healing*. 1963. Emmaus. PA: Rodale Press

Hutchens, A.R. 1969. *Indian Herbalogy of North America*. Windsor, Ontario: Merco Press

2 Sgoutas, D. and Kummerow, F.A. 1970. *American Journal of Clinical Nutrition* 23:1111

3 *Dairy Council Digest* 46:6 (Nov.-Dec. 1975)

4 White, A. et al. 1978. *Principles of Biochemistry*, 6th ed. New York: McGraw-Hill, p. 643

5 *Ibid.*, p. 641

6 *Ibid.*, p. 643

7 *Ibid.*, p. 644

8 Horrobin, D.F. 1980. *Medical Hypotheses* 6:785-800

9 Bierenbaum, M.L. and Oudhof, J.H. Abstract Book, International Prostaglandin Conference, Washington, D.C., May 1979, p. 10

10 Horrobin, David F. Private communication

11 Ibid

12 McCormick, J. N. et al. 1977. *Lancet* 2:508

13 Oster, P. et al. *Research in Experimental Medicine* (Berlin) 175:287-291

14 Vaddadi, K.S. and Horrobin, D.F. 1979 *Journal of Medical Science* 7:52

15 Passwater, Richard A. 1980. *The Easy No-Flab Diet*. New York: Marek Publishers

16 Passwater, Richard A. 1978. *Cancer and Its Nutritional Therapies.* New Canaan, CT: Keats Publishing, Inc.
17 Passwater, Richard A. 1980. *Selenium as Food and Medicine.* New Canaan, CT: Keats Publishing, Inc.
18 Horrobin, D. F. et al. 1979. *Medical Hypotheses* 5:969-985
19 Horrobin, D.F. et al. 1980. *Medical Hypotheses* 6:469-486
20 Dunbar, L.M. and Bailey, J. M. 1975. *Journal of Biology and Chemistry* 250:1152-1154
21 Bailey, J.M. 1977. *Lipid Metabolism in Mammals* (2) New York: Plenum Press
22 Puck, T.T. 1977. *Proceedings of the National Academy of Science* 74:4491-4495
23 Johnson, G.S. et al. 1975. *Proceedings of the National Academy of Science* 68:425-429
24 Horrobin, David F. Private communication
25 Houtsmuller, A.J. et al. 1980. *Nutritional Metabolism* 24:105-118
26 Horrobin, D.F. and Cunnane, S.C. 1980. *Medical Hypotheses* 6:277-296
27 Horrobin, D.F. and Manku, M.S. 1980. *British Medical Journal* 280:1363-1366
28 Horrobin, D.F. 1980. *Medical Hypotheses* 6:929-942
29 Horrobin, D.F. 1979. *Lancet* 529:531
30 Vaddadi, K.S. 1979. *Prostaglandins and Medicine* 2:77-80
31 Horrobin, D.F. Private communication